THE SUPER SIX WORKOUT

DISCOVER THE PROVEN BEST EXERCISES TO PACK ON SERIOUS MUSCLE MASS QUICKLY

By

SCOTT OTERI

Copyright © 2015

Table of Contents

INTRODUCTION

Back in the golden age of bodybuilding and strength training, before steroids, workout machines, functional training and all that other stuff became popular, men built muscle using barbells and their own bodyweight. Guys were as strong as they looked and they looked fantastic! Those classic physiques of yesteryear looked like Greek sculptures hewn out of granite.

Fast forward to today and not only have the physiques changed but so too have the training methods. Where squats and pull-ups were once workout mainstays, they are now often replaced with leg presses and lat pull downs. These movements might seem like they are the same but they really aren't and the lack of strength and muscle all too common in today's gyms is testament to the ineffectiveness of many of the exercises modern trainees build their workouts upon.

Good old barbell exercises are hard work but that's why they produce the best results. The old school guys knew this but, over the years, hard work has fallen out of fashion and all too many wannabe strength trainers have been seduced by the siren's song of exercise machines and easy workouts, subsequently failing to get meaningful results from their training.

Barbell exercises, like those that feature in this book, are more than just a way to build muscle; they also develop real-world strength and athleticism, develop skill and coordination and could even be said to build courage and character.

Why are these exercises so beneficial? Good question!

Barbell exercises are, by and large, compound in nature which simply means they involve multiple muscles and joints at the same time. Squats, for example, use not only every muscle in your lower body but virtually every muscle in your upper body to. Compared to the leg extension, leg curl or even the leg press, squats are a much more valuable, productive and effective exercise simply because they make you work harder.

Additionally, compound exercises like squats and deadlifts trigger a cascade of anabolic hormones – anabolic hormones being essential for muscle and strength building. These simple but never easy barbell exercises trigger the "grow or die" response that helped keep our ancestors from becoming extinct.

A brutally hard set of squats, for example, has been shown to significantly elevate both growth hormone AND testosterone production as well as increasing insulin sensitivity. This holy trinity of hormones is essential for building muscle and burning fat. Triceps kick and leg curls won't produce the same results.

Another factor to consider is that barbell exercises generally allow you to lift the greatest amount of weight and when it comes to building muscle and strength, the more weight the better. Which do you think will build the biggest, strongest pecs; flyes using a pair of 20kg dumbbells or bench pressing with 100kg? The answer should be pretty obvious!

Barbell exercises are also arguably more functional than the exercises that many trainers label as such. Squats with a heavy barbell or deadlifts will prepare your body for virtually every demanding task you are ever likely to face. Single leg squats on a BOSU ball? The only thing that will help you do is get a job in a circus – as a clown!

The fitness industry is a big and ever growing business which depends on reinventing the wheel over and over again so that gym owners and gym users continue to spend more and more money. Manufacturers produce machines that gym owners buy and therefore must encourage gym members to use. At no point are the results you are likely to experience part of the equation.

In contrast, barbells and weight plates are relatively cheap, take up very little space, don't require expensive sales strategies and are often viewed as old fashioned and yet, these inert pieces of iron will get you the body you want in much less time than any conceivable combination of expensive, complicated, expansive exercise machines ever will.

So, get ready to turn your back on much of what the fitness industry currently has to offer and embrace the old school way to building muscle and strength. You'll probably be surprised and even little sceptical that such a simple selection of exercises and uncomplicated workouts will deliver such great results but if what you are currently doing isn't working, what have you got to lose? The answer, of course, is nothing but you have everything to gain and remember; there is no school like old school!

The Super Six Workout programme

The Super Six workout is so called because it is built around six compound and highly effective exercises; the squat, bench press and bent over row, the deadlift, overhead press and pull-up. Between them, these six exercises work each and every major muscle in your body and will develop strength far better than any of the other exercises currently in vogue in many gyms.

These simple (but not easy!) exercises are as old as strength training itself and the reason they have stood the test of time is that they will work for anyone who has the patience and dedication to focus on them. And don't worry if you aren't sure how to perform these fabulous exercises, there are detailed instructions in the next few chapters.

It's all but guaranteed that if you work up to squatting double your bodyweight and overhead pressing your bodyweight you will be not only very strong but very big too. Achieving such standards will be hard and it will take time but the destination makes the journey worthwhile and you'll stand out from the crowd in virtually any gym as a result.

Programme variations…

There are several variations of the Super Six workout so you can pick and choose the option that suits you best. However, whichever variation you choose just remember to focus on the specified lifts and don't dilute your workouts by adding additional, usually unproductive exercises, that will detract from your progress and rob you of energy that would be better spent on the key exercises.

Option one – great for beginners or busy people		
	Monday	**Thursday**
1	Squats	Deadlifts
2	Bench Press	Overhead Press

3	Bent Over Rows	Pull-ups

Option two – the best option for the majority of exercisers				
		Monday	Wednesday	Friday
Week 1	1	Squats	Deadlifts	Squats
	2	Bench Press	Overhead Press	Bench Press
	3	Bent Over Rows	Pull-ups	Bent Over Rows
Week 2	1	Deadlifts	Squats	Deadlifts
	2	Overhead Press	Bench Press	Overhead Press
	3	Pull-ups	Bent Over Rows	Pull-ups

Option three – ideal if you only have time for short workouts				
	Monday	Tuesday	Thursday	Friday
1	Squats	Bench Press	Deadlifts	Overhead Press
2		Bent Over Rows		Pull-ups

Sets, reps and rest periods

It's not enough to build a programme around the best exercises; you also need to consider the number of sets and reps you perform and also how long you rest between sets too. Again, there are several options to choose from. Bottom line; so long as you work hard, strive to increase your weights week by week, eat healthily and plentifully and get sufficient sleep, you WILL get stronger and build muscle.

		Rest between sets
Option one	Three sets of eight reps	90 – 120 seconds
Option two	Four sets of twelve reps	60 – 90 seconds

Option three	Five sets of five reps	120 – 180 seconds
Option four	Six sets of four reps	120 – 180 seconds
Option five	Eight sets of three reps	90 – 120 seconds
Option six	10, 8, 6, 6, 6 reps	60 – 120 seconds

The last rep of each set should be hard but still completable in good form. You should feel that you have one or maybe two reps left in the tank at the end of your set. Leaving this margin ensures that you'll be able to increase the weight next time – even if it's only by a single kilo or even less.

A note about pull-ups

If you can't do bodyweight pull-ups, use one of the alternatives described in the pull-up chapter until you can. Once you are able to knock them out like a pro, increase your bodyweight by wearing a weighted vest or back pack to make this tremendous back builder more effective. Alternatively, if you prefer, do as many reps as you can per set with just your bodyweight. Either way, so long as you use more weight OR do more reps, you will get stronger.

What; no arms, abs or calves?

You've probably noticed that there are no biceps curls, triceps kickbacks or calf raises in this programme. This is NOT an oversight but a deliberate planning decision. There is nothing inherently wrong with these exercises but the muscles that they target, especially the arm, will get all the stimulation they need from the specified exercises in each programme.

For example, which muscle do you think will fail first when you are doing bench presses or overhead presses? The answer is the triceps. Doing additional triceps work will merely add insult to injury and may even limit your performance in your next workout. The same is true of the biceps and their involvement in pull-ups and bent over rows. Doing more exercise volume than you actually need to build muscle and strength simply delays the recovery process and means you'll be less able to work at your maximum next time.

As for abs, what do you think are holding your spine in proper alignment when you squat and deadlift? Yep – it's your abs. By all means do a couple of sets of abs after your main exercises are finished but don't go thinking that they'll make any real difference to your ab development; the hard work has already been done when you were squatting and deadlifting.

As for your lower legs, your calves also get a great workout when you squat and deadlift; they work really hard to ensure you don't fall forward onto your toes. If you have "chicken-calves" then feel free to add a few sets of single leg standing calf raises to the end of each workout. Why this exercise in particular? Because it's the best calf-builder by far!

Putting it all together

So, choose your programme option and then decide on which set and rep scheme you want to use. Select a weight that means the last rep of each set is challenging (this may take some experimentation but you'll get it in the end) and then strive to add a little more weight to the bar each and every workout. When you hit a plateau and cannot add any more weight, simply switch to a different set/rep scheme and start over. Deceptively simple, devastatingly effective; work hard and you WILL see results.

Warming up and cooling down

Before each and every workout, make sure you spend a few minutes preparing your body and mind for what is to come. This is best achieved by doing a few minutes of light cardio, performing a handful of dynamic stretches like leg swings and arm circles and then doing a couple of progressively heavier sets of the exercises you are about to perform.

For example, if you are doing five sets of five reps with 80kg, warm up by doing ten reps with the empty 20kg bar, six reps with 40kg and then four reps with 60kg. That way you'll be ready for your 80kg but won't feel tired. The heavier the weight you'll be lifting, the more warm up sets you need so don't worry if you need five warm up sets for squats but only two for overhead presses.

On completion of your last set, spend a few more minutes gently stretching the muscles you have just been working, This will minimize muscle soreness and help keep your muscles flexible – an essential part of performing exercise like squats and bent over rows properly.

So then, and without further ado, turn the page and find out how to perform the Super Six exercises properly…

Exercise Catalog

Squat

The squatting movement pattern is one of the most common physical challenges you face on a day to day basis. Sitting down in a chair, getting off your bed, sitting on the loo and getting out of your car are all examples of the squat. In this chapter, you will learn how to squat properly and safely so that you can enjoy all the benefits this exercise has to offer.

If you look at a child when he/she squats down on the floor to play with toys you'll probably see a perfect squat in action. Their feet will be wide with the weight balanced evenly between forefoot and heel, their head and chest will be lifted, knees bent well past 90 degrees with the spine completely neutral. Ask an adult to perform the same movement and, in most cases, you'll be deafened by creaking knees and general groans of discomfort! So what has changed? Simply, as we age, our joints become less mobile and we adapt to sitting on chairs rather than sitting on our haunches. We basically lose our squat.

Losing your squat is a shame. Not only do you have to constantly look for chairs to sit on but we also rob ourselves of one of the most beneficial exercises that you can perform. Squatting well isn't easy however, when it comes to positive carryover to everyday activities and sporting performance, the squat is a "must do" for pretty much everyone. Whether you are a granny who wants to live an independent life or an Olympic gymnast looking to improve your vertical jump, you gotta squat!

Squat Anatomy

The squat, both the exercise and the movement pattern, uses just about every muscle in your lower body as well as many on your upper body. If you are short of time and can only perform one exercise in your workout, the barbell back squat is the logical choice. Squats work your calves, albeit indirectly, your hamstrings, quadriceps, abductors and adductors (outer and inner thighs respectively), your glutes, core and upper back. When the weights get heavy enough, squats also challenge your arms and shoulders too.

Squat Equipment

Squatting is best performed in a specially designed squat or power rack. This saves you having to clean and jerk the bar into place. In the old days, lifters used to stand the bar on its end and then roll it across their shoulders; a practice that is hard to recommend! A power rack also limits the extent of your downward travel so, if you are unfortunate enough to get stuck at the bottom of a squat, you can simply dump the bar on the catching rods and walk away.

Clothing wise, you'll need a T shirt that covers your upper back. While a back-revealing tank top may look terrific, you don't want the bar to slip while you lift and a more modest T shirt will help. For lower body wear, whether you choose long or short legged attire, make sure it is loose enough around your hips and bum to allow you to squat down in comfort. Busting the back out of your shorts is funny when it happens to someone else but not so funny when it happens to you, as many tight-pant-wearing exercisers find out to their cost.

Finally, your choice of shoe is very important. Ideally, you want a shoe with a thin, hard sole and a non-compressible heel. Weight lifting shoes have wooden soles and heels but unless you are going to lift very seriously, you don't need these. Spongy-soled running shoes will compress when the weights begin to get heavy and this added instability will not help you to squat well. In a pinch, and if your gym allows it, lifting in just your socks is better than spongy running shoes; just watch your toes.

As you'll be gripping the bar tightly, lifting chalk can be beneficial; chalk your hands and the centre of the bar to minimize the risk of any slippage. This is not essential but do make sure you dry your hands and upper back if you are a heavy sweater.

Squatting Technique

Chances are, if you squat down to sit in a chair or perform a similar squatting movement, you don't even think about how to do it. Strangely, as soon as there is a barbell on your shoulders, it's likely that your natural squatting instincts are all but forgotten and what should be a relatively simple movement becomes a real test of coordination and control. Don't worry, this is quite normal and is caused by the fact you are lifting a weight using your legs only when your body is hardwired to lift with your arms.

Set the barbell in the squat rack at mid-chest level. Too high and you'll have to rise up on tip toes to walk it out the rack. Too low and you'll have to squat it up and out of the rack, wasting precious energy. Grab the bar with an overhand slightly wider than shoulder-width grip. Wrap your thumbs around the bar and hold it tight. Duck under the bar and position your upper back under the bar. Make sure the bar is not resting on your neck but is low across your shoulders. This position should negate the need to pad the bar in any way. If it hurts your neck, the bar is too high.

Inhale, lift your chest and pull the bar firmly down onto your upper back. Try to keep your wrists straight and your elbows pushed slightly forwards. Stand up and un-rack the bar. Take a step back so you are clear of the catching hooks. Place your feet at least shoulder-width apart. The taller you are, the wider your feet will need to be. Turn your feet out slightly to they are set to a "five to one" position. Lift your chest again and inhale deeply. Reset your upper back so that your entire upper body feels tight. You are now ready to squat!

Initiate your descent by pushing your hips backwards. As your hips move back, bend your knees and try to push your knees apart. Imagine you are trying to spread the floor with your feet. Keep your chest up, your upper body tight and your core braced. Descend until your thighs are parallel to the floor. To check this, your hip crease should be level with your knees.

Keep your lower back tightly arched and never rounded. Imagine you are trying to squat down between your feet. Don't pause at the bottom but, instead, make the transition from downward movement to upward movement dynamic and strong. Push your hips upwards, drive down through your feet, keep your chest up and extend your knees. Do not lift your head as this will simply rob you of much of your pushing power. Stand all the way up until you are back in the starting position and then repeat.

Perform your set and then walk back into the squat rack and replace the bar.

It is common practice when squatting to inhale as you descend and then exhale as you ascend. This is fine until the weight begins to get heavy. Once you are lifting more substantial weights it will become necessary to breathe between repetitions as exhaling will reduce the intra-abdominal pressure necessary for lumbar support. For now though, just remember to keep breathing.

Squat Faults

Nobody likes ugly squats – they are less beneficial and also increase your risk of injury. You might not even realise you have an ugly squat unless you film yourself or have access to an experienced coaches' assessment. Here are a few common squat faults and how to fix them...

- Rounded lower back at the bottom – This is most commonly associated with deep squatting. If your hamstrings are tight or your feet are placed too close together, your pelvis may be pulled under which results in a rounded lower back. Make sure your hamstrings are sufficiently flexible, move your feet slightly wider and also reduce the depth of your squat to where you can maintain a strong lumbar arch. Rounding of the lower back can also be a sign of weak core and spinal erectors. In this case, reduce the weight on the bar until your core is able to support the efforts of your legs. Finally, remember to initiate the movement by pushing your hips back – this often cures most rounded back problems.

- Weight shifts onto your toes – Make sure you can wiggle your toes inside your shoes before you start your descent. Also, focus on pushing your hips back BEFORE you bend your knees. Placing the bar across your neck rather than your upper back can also contribute to a forward weight shift so make sure the bar is placed low across your shoulders. Finally, your lower back/core may be weak and struggling to support the weight. This can result in excessive forward lean and push the weight onto your toes.

- Knees track inwards/outwards – Hip instability can result in inward/outward tracking of your knees. Firstly, remember to push your knees outward and try to spread the floor with your feet. You should do this in the setup, descent and ascent. Secondly, try stretching your adductors or inner thigh muscles so that they are less likely to pull your knees inwards. Finally, strengthen your hip abductors or outer hip/thigh muscles by performing lying side leg lifts and hip abductions using a resistance band. Sidesteps with a resistance band around your knees is also an effective way to strengthen your abductors.

Squat variations

While the barbell back squat, as described above, is probably the ultimate form of squatting, there are a few variations worth mentioning. For those of you new to performing this king of exercises, get to grips with the bodyweight squat before progressing onto the full barbell squat.

The front squat is favoured by many athletes and by Olympic weight lifters and involves racking the bar across the front of your shoulders instead of the back. This results in a more upright torso and a greater range of movement at the knee joint. This makes the front squat a more quad dominant exercise compared to the back squat. Many coaches believe that this means the front squat has greater carryover to jumping activities. The more upright torso and reduction of hip musculature recruitment means that front squatters generally use lighter weights than back squatters but the reduced load on the lumbar muscles may be beneficial for some exercisers. On the downside, the front squat can be uncomfortable if you have underdeveloped or lightly muscled shoulders or lack upper body flexibility.

Overhead squats are often used as functional movement screening test as your performance of this challenging exercise will reveal where your muscles are tight and/or weak. Overhead squatting usually uses the lightest loads but is still a very challenging exercise. If lower body strength is your goal, the overhead squat is probably not the best exercise to perform but if your aim is to improve mobility and flexibility, the overhead squat is an excellent choice. Performing overhead squats in your warm up can make back squats feel easy by comparison.

Hip belt squats provide a great option if you really don't like having a heavy weight resting on your shoulders or upper back. By slinging the weight low between your legs, your centre of gravity is moved downwards so balancing is easy and your lower back is completely unloaded. This leaves you free to concentrate on working your legs to the maximum. Hip belt squats are also a good option if you don't have access to a squat or power rack. On the downside, set up can be tricky and you'll need a well-padded hip belt and sturdy boxes for the performance of this exercise.

Remember; if you really want to develop strong, muscular and athletic legs, you really need to squat hard, deep, heavy and often! No, it won't be easy but then easy never gets you anything worthwhile.

Bench press

The barbell flat bench press, from this point onward referred to simply as the bench press, is one of the most commonly performed exercises in gyms today. Considered as one of the standard tests of strength, on discovering that you lift weights, many people will want to know "how much can you bench?" As well as being a popular exercise, the bench press is also one of the lifts contested in the sport of powerlifting.

The bench press is a relative newcomer as prior to the 1930's any pressing was performed either from a standing position or while lying on the floor – the so-called floor press. The subsequent advent of mass produced exercise benches resulted in the bench press becoming the popular and well known exercise it is today. It seems that, amongst young men at least, Monday is National Bench Press Day – something that won't be changing anytime soon!

As the bench press is so popular, it's only right that you learn to do it properly because good technique can make the difference between getting a lot of benefits from this seemingly simple exercise and permanently damaging your shoulders...

Bench Press Anatomy

The bench press is a horizontal pushing exercise and, as such, targets the majority of your upper body pushing muscles. While hand position and the slope of the bench you are using can alter the degree of stress placed on the various pushing muscles, in general, all variations of the bench press target the same muscles:

- Pectoralis major – pecs for short, these muscles make up the majority of your chest mass and are considered to be the agonists or prime movers in the bench press

- Anterior deltoids – located on the front of your shoulders, the anterior deltoids work with your pecs to flex your shoulder as you drive the bar off your chest
- Triceps brachii – the muscles on the back of your arm, commonly referred to simply as triceps, are responsible for extending your elbows

In addition to these structures, the muscles of your core, upper back and deep shoulders and even the legs also work very hard to ensure you have a stable base from which to push.

Bench Press Equipment

To perform the bench press safely, you need a bench press bench with built in uprights, an appropriate barbell, weight collars and a competent spotter. If you don't have a spotter, you can also perform the bench press in a power rack for safety. If you don't have a spotter or a power rack, perform dumbbell bench presses instead as getting pinned across the chest by a heavy barbell can result in severe injury.

Clothing-wise, anything that allows free and unrestricted movement of your shoulders and arms is fine. Unlike the squat and deadlift where footwear is important, you can pretty much wear whatever shoes you like for bench press but flat-soled shoes will provide a more positive connection to the floor. If you are a heavy sweater, you might benefit from wearing a T-shirt as opposed to a tank top or crop top so that your upper back does not slip and slide on the bench. As a courtesy to other gym users, place a sweat towel placed on the bench so minimize any sweat swapping!

Your grip in the bar is very important in the bench press so it may be worth considering the use of lifting chalk so your hands stay nice and dry. If your gym does not allow you to use chalk, make sure your hands and the bar are as dry as possible by wiping them both with the for mentioned sweat towel.

Bench Press Technique

For such a seemingly simple exercise, the bench press is actually quite a technical lift – especially if you want to avoid short and long term shoulder, elbow and wrist injuries while lifting the heaviest weights you can safely manage. Like all exercises, getting into the right position from the start will greatly increase your chances of performing the bench press properly.

With the barbell supported by the catching hooks on your bench, lie down so that your eyes are directly beneath the bar.

Place your feet flat on the floor so that your shins are vertical and your feet are wider than shoulder-width apart. This foot position will help make you more stable and thus better able to press the weight without any undue wobbling. Push your toes into the fronts of your shoes to activate the muscles in your legs and press your feet down into the floor. Although the bench press is an upper body exercise, you'll be using your entire body to brace your torso in position.

With your legs braced, keep your butt pressed firmly into the bench and then arch your lower back. A strong arch will help raise your chest toward the ceiling and subsequently reduce the distance the bar has to travel. Press your upper back firmly into the bench and shrug your shoulder blades back and down. By activating your upper back muscles, you provide a rock-steady platform from which to work.

Reach up and grasp the bar. You should only need to lift the bar a few inches to take it clear of the hooks. Your hands should be slightly wider than shoulder width apart so that, at the bottom of the movement, your forearms are vertical. Wrap your fingers and thumbs around the bar and grip it tightly. Do not use a thumb-less grip as it increases your risk of dropping the bar. Gripping the bar tightly will activate the muscles in your forearms that stabilize your wrists – imagine you are trying to leave fingerprints in the bar! Also, try to rotate your hands outward. Although impossible, this action helps fire up your lats which provide a shelf of support for your shoulders.

Un-rack the bar and then hold it directly over your shoulders. Reinforce your lower back arch and shoulders and remember to press your feet down intro the floor. Note the position of the bar in relation to the ceiling – this is your start and finish position for each and every repetition. Make a conscious effort to return the bar to this spot at the end of each rep. Take a big breath in.

Bend your arms and lower the bar down toward the highest point of your chest. The descent of the bar should be controlled but not super-slow. As you lower the bar, your elbows should tuck slightly down and in towards your torso. This slight elbow tucking action takes stress off of your shoulders. It is not a good idea to keep your upper arms out at 90 degrees to your body. Although this may slightly increase the involvement of your pecs, it places your shoulders in a mechanically disadvantageous position which can lead to both short-term and long-term injuries.

Let the bar lightly touch your chest. Imagine there is a plate of glass resting on your chest and while you want to touch it, you mustn't break it. Without pausing, drive the bar up and off your chest. Try to lift the bar faster than you lowered it. As the weights get heavier this will become impossible but if you try to do this, you are less likely to get stuck with the bar across your chest. Push the bar all the way back up to the starting position and then exhale. Inhale, reset your arch and upper back and perform another repetition.

The action of inhaling between reps performs a couple of functions. Firstly, by inflating your chest, you reduce the distance the bar has to travel which protects your shoulder joint from hyper-extension. Secondly, inhalation increases intra-abdominal pressure which helps keep your spine stable.

While the bench is supporting your body, intra-abdominal pressure supports your spine and ensures that the tension in your legs and force generated by your arms are not "lost" in your midsection.

On completion of your set and with the weight held over your chest and arms fully extended, push the bar back to the catching hooks. Do not try to complete your least rep and simultaneously push the bar back onto the hooks. If you fail to lock out your arms you may miss the hooks and be in the unenviable position of having a barbell crashing down towards your forehead. Press up, lock out and then re-rack.

Bench Press Faults

The main problems associated with poor bench press performance come from failing to set up correctly and then trying to lift too much weight. If you always place your feet flat, activate your leg muscles, arch your lower back, lift your chest and pull your shoulders down and back you should have little trouble performing picture-perfect bench presses. That being said, watch out for the following...

- No lower back arch - this is normally seen in people who perform the bench press with their feet elevated. Don't do this! Lack of back arch encourages the shoulders to round forwards and also robs you of essential shoulder stability. If you can't comfortably plant your feet flat on the floor, the bench is too high. Raise the level of the floor by stacking some weight plates or use the top of a step box but make sure that you are still able to create a strong lower back arch.
- Wrists bend back – over extended wrists indicate that you aren't gripping the bar hard enough and you are holding the bar too high in your hand. The bar should sit in the bottom of your hand. If you get to the point where you are lifting very heavy weights, you may want

to consider using wrist wraps but for now, focus on developing good "raw" technique. Straight wrists are strong wrists.

- Uneven bar – make sure that your hands are placed equidistant from the centre of the bar – use the knurled rings to check your position. It is very common for one arm to be stronger than the other and this can manifest in the bar being tilted. If you do have a left to right strength imbalance, place all of your mental effort on your weak arm. Use your mind to help your weaker side. Your stronger arm will carry on regardless. After a while, you should find your imbalance fixes itself.

Bench Press Variations

While the barbell version of this exercise is by far and away the most common form of bench pressing, there are a number of notable alternatives. Altering the incline of the bench places an increased demand on different parts of the pectoralis major. Incline bench presses shift the emphasis onto the clavicular or upper part of the chest while decline bench presses target the lower or sternal aspect. For strength, the flat bench press is best but if you specifically want to develop your chest for aesthetic reasons, using different bench angles can change the shape of your chest muscles.

Dumbbell bench presses add an extra stability and balance demand and makes the exercise harder. As you have to control two weights and not just one, left to right strength imbalances can be spotted and addressed. Dumbbell bench pressing also allows for a less restrictive shoulder movement which may provide a more comfortable workout if you have already got sore shoulders.

For an even greater balance challenge, dumbbell bench presses can also be performed using a stability ball but make sure that the ball you are using is marked as "anti burst" and rated for strength. Not all balls are up to the task.

Narrow grip bench presses involve shifting your hands in to a shoulder-width grip increase the range of movement at your elbows and therefore increases triceps involvement. The so-called narrow grip bench press is an excellent triceps building exercise and useful if you have trouble locking out the bar at the end of a repetition of regular bench presses.

Single arm dumbbell bench presses are a great way to address left to right strength imbalances and also a champion core exercise. Your abs must work very hard to keep your body from twisting. This is a great exercise for boxers, martial artists and rugby players.

So, the next time National Bench Press Day rolls around, you'll be lifting like a pro and safe in the knowledge you are performing this popular, chest-building exercise safely and effectively. And while the Smith machine may seem like an attractive and safe way to perform bench presses, the fixed path of the bar places an unnatural stress on your shoulders and so this exercise variation is best avoided.

Bent over row

The bent over row is one of the most controversial exercises around. Much of this controversy stems from the fact that it's a technically demanding exercise that, if performed badly, could result in back injury. For many years, it was considered as a vital movement and many lifters, both bodybuilders and Olympic lifters, hoisted huge weights in this exercise but since the advent of machines offering a seemingly similar and potentially safer alternative, the bent over row has fallen out of favour in many circles. This is a shame because, as exercises go, you won't find many that are as effective or beneficial.

The main perceived problem with the bent over row is the position in which it is performed – no prizes for guessing it involves bending over! Many people, when asked to perform this simple and often common task, bend over from the waist which results in a rounded back that would make a camel proud. This rounded back position, especially when loaded, can cause irrefutable damage to your back but, as we won't be performing a bent over row in that fashion, this risk is all but eliminated. The key to a good, safe bent over row is bending from the hips – something commonly referred to as hip hinging.

One of the problems in exercise is that many exercises that are deemed dangerous are only dangerous when performed with poor technique. The deadlift is a notorious back-breaker of an exercise and this is true IF you lift with a rounded back. If, however, you lift with a solid lower back arch and strongly braced abdominals, it is possible to lift very substantial weights in absolute safety. The squat is often labelled as bad for your knees which is true if you dive-bomb into the bottom position of the squat and bounce out of the hole using the elastic properties of your knee joints. Needless to say, if you have read the previous chapter on how to deadlift and squat properly you won't do either. Most exercises are safe to perform provided you perform the exercise properly, with control and using appropriate loading. The bent over row is no exception.

Bent over row anatomy

There are two distinct ways to perform the bent over row – using a wider-than shoulder width grip and a narrow grip. While performance is similar, each variation works your muscles in a different way. As such, you should treat the wide grip and narrow grip variations of the bent over row as completely different exercises and choose one or the other according to your goals.

As the Super Six workout programme also includes pull-ups, a terrific lat exercise, you would do well to focus on the wide grip version as it works a different area of your back. For that reason, we'll introduce that variation first...

Wide grip bent over rows

The wide grip bent over row, WGBOR form here on, targets the muscles across the back of your shoulders and between your shoulder blades, specifically your posterior deltoids, middle fibres of trapezius and rhomboids. Holding your spine in a neutral position is the job of your erector spinae and obviously your hips and legs are also involved in maintaining your stance. In addition, your biceps brachii on the front of your upper arms and your forearm flexor muscles are also strongly involved in bending your arms and gripping the bar respectively.

Narrow grip bent over rows

The narrow grip bent over row, NGBOR from here on, works many of the muscles described above but places an additional emphasis on your latissimus dorsi muscles, lats for short, on the side of your upper back.

In simple terms, the WGBOR is more of a mid-back postural exercise while the NGBOR is an effective lat builder. Both involve your arms, lower back and legs to more or less the same degree.

Bent over row equipment

The bent over row can be performed using dumbbells, a Powerbag, kettlebells or even a heavy rock but for ease of explanation, in this article we'll focus on the barbell version of the exercise.

Other than a barbell, you don't really need any specialist equipment for this particular exercise. You may find getting into your starting position is a little easier if you place your bar in a waist-high power rack or on blocks put this is purely optional. As you will be gripping the bar, you might benefit from using some lifting chalk or having a hand towel nearby to keep your hands dry but the knurling on the bar should ensure a good grip.

Speaking of grip, some lifters use straps to help them attach themselves to the bar. While this is an effective strategy, it can lead to problems in the long term. Firstly, your grip never improves as you are ignoring the symptom of weak gripping muscles and not addressing the cause. Secondly, your grip is a built in safety device that limits how much weight you can effectively lift. If you can't hold something with your hands, your back probably won't be able to support it either we don't recommend you use them unless your grip is really poor. If that's the case, spend some time beefing up your grip!

Shoes are less of an issue than they were in squats and deadlifts but as this exercise is performed in a standing position, firm shoes with a flat sole are going to be better than spongy running shoes that distort when loaded with extra weight. This is not a deal breaker though.

Bent over row technique

As mentioned earlier, there are two distinct variations of the bent over row: the wide grip and the narrow grip. To perform the wide grip bent over row, position your hands at approximately the same distance apart as you would use for the bench press, discussed back in the previous chapter. Use a pronated or palms-down grip and wrap your thumbs tightly around the bar to provide the best purchase possible. For the narrow grip bent over row, grasp the bar with a supinated or palms-up hip-width grip. This position is best for targeting your lats and maximizing the pulling power of your biceps.

Once you have decided which bent over row you are going to perform, the exercises are pretty similar.

Firstly, grasp a barbell with the appropriate grip – wide and overhand to target your upper-mid back and narrow and underhand to focus more on your lats. Stand with your feet between shoulder and hip width-apart and bend your knees slightly. Pull your shoulders down and back, lift your chest and inhale.

From this position, hinge forwards from your hips. As you lean forwards keep your chest up, your weight on your heels and maintain your lower back arch. If you find your lower back is rounding out, bend your knees a little more to put a little more slack in your hamstrings.

Ideally you want to incline your body so your torso is slightly above parallel to the floor i.e. your head is slightly above your hips. Your ultimate back position will be dictated by the length of your hamstrings but above all, remember that your lower back should never become rounded. If you are unable to lean forwards while maintaining your lumbar curve, you will be better off using one of the alternatives discussed below. Remember that your neck is part of your spine so it is important you keep your chin tucked in and avoid looking at yourself in the mirror. Raising your head will affect the position of your lumbar spine. If you do want to look at yourself in the mirror (you handsome devil you!) lift your eyes and not your whole head.

Let the weight hang straight down from your shoulders. If the bar is heavy enough this will happen automatically but if you are using a light weight, you may need to check this in the mirror. Your arms should be perfectly vertical in relation to the floor.

From this position initiate your pull by thinking about drawing your elbows behind you. Imagine your arms are merely cables that connect the weight to your back muscles. In the WGBOR, pull the bar up and into your chest so it touches in the same place as the barbell bench press. For the NGBOR, pull the bar up and into your bellybutton or slightly lower. Irrespective of which version you are performing, keep your body as still as possible and focus on driving your elbows back – really squeeze them together!

Pause for a split second with the bar touching your chest or abdomen as appropriate and then slowly extend your arms to return to the starting position. Inhale as you pull the bar up and exhale as you lower it. Do not relax between repetitions as this can lead to problems when you progress to a heavier load. Keep your shoulders and core braced, make sure your chest remains elevated and your lower back slightly arched. For both versions of the BOR, your body is the bench which provides the stable platform for your arms to work from.

Unlike many exercises that can be safely performed to muscular failure, the bent over row should only be performed to form failure i.e. the point at which your technique starts to break down. Don't cheat the bar up by jerking with your arms, legs or back – this is a quick route to injury.

Bent over row faults

The BOR is quite a complex movement – mainly because it involves pretty much all of your body. There are a few common faults to look out for...

- Bent wrists – in an effort to get the bar to touch the chest or abdomen, some exercisers will shorten the distance the bar has to travel by bending their wrists under. This places a lot of stress on the wrists and also detracts from the exercise in general. Focus on leading with your elbows and don't worry if the bar fails to touch your chest or abdomen. Tight chest muscles or long limbs may make this difficult.
- Rounded lower back – to be avoided at all costs, a rounded lower back may indicate tight hamstrings and/or hip flexors, a weakness in the glutes or erector spinae or general lack of body awareness. Try bending your knees slightly to slacken off your hamstrings and performing static stretches for your hamstrings and hip flexors. To train your body to recognise the correct position for the BOR, before you do a set lie on your front on the floor with your shoulders and elbows flexed to 90 degrees. From this position, lift your head, chest and shoulders off the floor using the strength of your lower back. Squeeze your shoulders back and hold this position for 20 to 30 seconds. Relax, rest a moment and then get into your BOR starting position trying to replicate the sensation of using your back muscles for support.

Bent over row variations

While the basic barbell version of this exercise is a fantastic back builder, variety is, as they say, the spice of life so why not try these variations once you have mastered the basic barbell versions described above? All versions can be performed using a wide or narrow grip as appropriate.

The dead-stop barbell row is sometimes called a Pendlay row after Olympic weight lifting coach Glenn Pendlay, this version begins with the barbell on the floor. With the barbell at your feet, bend forwards in good form and grasp the bar with the appropriate grip. Then, with your core braced, pull the bar up and in to touch your body. Lower it back down to the floor and allow the weight to rest momentarily before repeating. By starting from a dead-stop each time, you eliminate much of the elastic energy stored in your muscles. This makes the exercise harder and promotes an increase in strength at the beginning of the pull. This rowing variation requires great hamstring flexibility and a very strong core.

The single armed dumbbell bent over row is a popular exercise that allows you to lift heavy weights as your spare arm is used to provide extra support for your spine. Be aware though that just because your free arm is providing some extra support, you must still endeavour to maintain good postural alignment. Rounding your back when it is under load is NEVER a good idea! You can perform this exercise with both feet on the floor or with one knee resting on a bench. Whichever you choose, your back should be in exactly the same position with your hips squared and level.

Two point single arm bent over rows increase the rotational demands placed on your core. Using one dumbbell instead of two and standing in an unsupported position means that your body will naturally want to rotate towards the weighted side. Despite using one weight, your torso should look exactly the same as though you were using two: chest lifted, lower back arched, shoulders level and hips squared. Place your free hand on your lower back to monitor your lumbar curve.

The one point single arm bent over row combines increased balance with the same anti-rotation qualities of the two point single arm bent over row. This exercise is very challenging but the added complexity comes at the cost of limiting the amount of weight you can use. A great option if you only have limited weight available or prefer to make your workouts more demanding by selecting technically challenging exercises. (Or want to join a circus!)

There is an old saying in training; if you want to GROW, you gotta ROW so make sure you work your rows just as hard as you work your bench presses. Big pecs are great but a big back will really get you attention and give you a serious look of power!

Deadlift

The deadlift has a chequered history. During the late 19th and early 20th centuries, it was known as the "health lift" as it had such a profound effect on total body strength and wellbeing. Fast forward to the era of strength training machines and sedentary lifestyles, the deadlift is now often considered a slightly dangerous exercise with many inherent risks. Yes, deadlifts are demanding and if performed badly may increase your risk of injury but this is not the fault of the exercise as much as it is the fault of incorrect instruction.

The deadlift is so-called because the weight if lifted from a dead stop. Not only is the deadlift a superior strength building exercise, it also mirrors the technique we should all use when picking just about anything off the floor; if you strength train, at some point you will have to perform a deadlift when you pick your weights up so you might as well learn to do it right!

Deadlift Anatomy

It's almost easier to list the muscles NOT used in a deadlift as this exercise is very much a whole body exercise. From your heels to the back of your neck via your arms, core and back – almost every muscle on your body is used when deadlifting. From bottom to top, the main muscles involved in the deadlift are:

- Gastrocnemius and soleus – calf muscles
- Hamstrings – rear of thigh
- Quadriceps – front of thigh
- Gluteus maximus – bottom muscles
- Erector spine – muscles on either side of your spine
- Core muscles – deep muscles surrounding your internal organs
- Rhomboids and trapezius – muscles of the upper back
- Latissimus dorsi – side upper back muscles

- Deltoids – muscles of the shoulder
- Biceps and triceps – front and back of the upper arm
- Forearm flexors – gripping muscles

In terms of workout economy, deadlifts get a lot of work done in a very short space of time. Add in a few sets of press-ups, dips or bench presses and you've covered just about every muscle in your body.

Deadlift Equipment

Theoretically, you can deadlift just about anything but for instructional purposes, we will be focusing on the barbell deadlift. To make the exercise as safe as possible, you will need to raise your barbell so that it is about 23 centimetres (9 inches) off the floor. You can either place it on a couple of sturdy boxes, some stacked weight plates or use Olympic sized lightweight training plates to achieve this. Once you are strong enough, you can simply use 20kg (45 pound) weight plates on the bar as these are the correct height. While you can deadlift with the bar closer to the ground, this is NOT recommended for most lifters as doing so encourages a rounded lower back.

Clothing-wise, make sure your leg wear allows you to bend forwards unrestricted. Many lifters burst the backside of their shorts when deadlifting so please learn by their embarrassing mistakes!

For footwear, initially any kind of athletic shoe will do but as you get more proficient, you'll find that shoes with little or no cushioning and low heels are best. Soft, spongy shoes are great for running and other high impact activities but for deadlifts, they simply compress and deform which can make you very unstable. Not something you want. Also, thick shoes mean you have to lift the weight further. This might not seem important right now but once you get to lifting serious weight, every inch matters.

Some lifters use chalk to help prevent grip problems. When learning the deadlift, this shouldn't be too much of an issue but you should still make sure your hands are as dry as possible before grabbing the bar. You can't lift what you can't hold!

Deadlift Technique

So – let's get ready to lift! With your barbell raised as described above stand in the middle of the bar. Move your feet so that they are around hip-width apart. Keep your feet parallel or, if preferred, turn them very slightly outward. The bar should be directly over the middle of your foot and around two inches from your shins. Lift your chest, arch your back slightly and pull your shoulders down and back. Remember this position as it is vital for successful deadlifting.

Lean forwards and grasp the bar with a shoulder-width overhand grip. This means your palms should be facing your legs. A wider grip is not recommended as it merely increases the distance you have to lift the weight. Wrap your hands tightly around your bar and put your thumb on top of your first two fingers. This reinforces your grip and prevents slippage.

With straight arms, lift your chest, arch your lower back, pull your shoulders down and back and lower your hips below shoulder-height. Angle your head so that you are looking at the floor around three meters (10 feet) in front of you. Take a big lung full of air and get ready for blast-off. Take the slack out of the bar so that your entire body feels coiled like a spring ready to explode. Brace your abs and you are ready to go.

Without bending your arms, extend your knees and hips simultaneously. As you break the bar away from the floor, drive your hips forwards, continue extending your knees and stand up. It is essential that your hips do not rise faster than your shoulders. This increases the distance between the weight and your base of support which essentially places a greater load on your spine. Ideally, your shoulders should rise faster than your hips or, at the very least, the same speed. At the top of the movement make sure your knees are locked out and your hips extended. Pause for a second and admire the view!

Lowering the weight is easy enough as gravity is now your friend but it is essential you put the weight down with good technique to minimize your risk of injury. With your arms still straight, chest lifted and shoulders pulled down and back, push your hips back slightly and then bend your knees. Pushing your hips back first means the bar will miss your knees as you lower it to the ground.

Control your descent or the weight but there is no need to go super-slow. Likewise, don't merely drop it either. When the bar touches down, reset your grip and back position and then repeat. Perform a set of five and then rest. If everything went well, add some weight and perform another set of five. Continue adding weight until your form starts to deteriorate. When this happens, go back a step in weight and perform another set or two of five. Make a note of this weight and use it next time.

Only increase the weight if you feel comfortable and your technique is solid. There is nothing wrong with staying with the same weight while you perfect your form.

Breathing

In general, you should inhale as lift the weight and then exhale as you lower it however, once the weight gets heavy and you are working in the lower rep ranges, you will find it necessary to breathe between reps. This breathing pattern increases intra-abdominal pressure and lumbar support but also increases blood pressure. If you have any blood pressure issues, use lighter weights for this exercise and follow the inhale/raise, exhale/lower pattern of breathing.

A Note on Grip

Many lifters choose to use what is known as a mixed grip where one hand faces forwards and one faces backwards. This generally allows the lifter to use more weight. On the down side, the supinated or forward facing hand places the biceps of that arm in a very stretched position which can lead to injury. Also, a mixed grip can result in shoulder and upper back imbalances. If you do choose to use a mixed grip. Try top alternate sides on a set by set basis or, better still, only use the mixed grip for your last and hardest set.

Deadlift Faults

Hopefully you will have performed a perfect set of deadlifts however; you may have experienced one or more of the following problems. Correct these faults early on in your deadlifting career as once you get into bad habits, they can be tough to fix.

- Rounded lower back – remember to keep your chest up and shoulders back. Keep the weight close to you and do not let your hips rise faster than your shoulders. You may also benefit from some specific lower back strengthening exercises.
- Falling forwards during the lift – make sure your weight is on your heels and that you can wiggle your toes inside your shoes at all times. Try deadlifting in shoes with a lower heel or, if your gym allows it, in bare feet.
- Fall backward at the top of the lift – don't lean back excessively at the top of the movement. Simply stand up straight with the weight held over your feet. No need to arch your back at the top.

Deadlift Variations

The barbell deadlift is probably one of the best exercises you can perform but there are a few variations you might want to consider learning for variation...

The Romanian deadlift is a hip-dominant movement where the knees remain slightly bent but rigid throughout the exercise. Romanian deadlifts are performed from the top down as opposed to the ground up which provides a unique stimulus for strength development.

Sumo deadlifts are, like regular deadlifts, performed from the ground up but utilize a very wide stance. In sumo deadlifts, your hands are inside your legs rather than outside. The idea of the sumo deadlift is that it reduces the distance the bar has to travel which means, in theory, you can lift more weight. Sumo deadlifts are used by power lifters and make a nice change from the regular version.

Trap bar deadlifts use a special bar where you stand directly between the weights as opposed to behind it. Trap bars allow you to keep a more upright body position but they really mimic the squat more than the deadlift.

Rack pulls are partial deadlifts performed from knee height to full extension. These are used by lifters who have trouble completing a deadlift due to weakness in the upper range of movement.

Conversely, **non-lockout deadlifts** involve lifting the bar from the ground and only raising it to knee height. This exercise variation can improve your ability to break the bar away from the floor. Both of these techniques are best left to more advanced lifters.

So now you know how to deadlift properly and safely. Remember, use the same technique regardless of whether you are lifting dumbbells of the ground before

doing a set of curls, picking your kids up for a cuddle or attempting to deadlift double your bodyweight! Deadlifts are THE safest way to lift.

Overhead press

Of all the upper body lifts, the overhead press is probably the most challenging, beneficial and functional exercise you can perform. While the bench press is often considered the king of the upper body lifts, when you press a weight above your head from a standing position, it's all about you, the bar and mean old gravity! There is no bench to support you, no semi-flexible sternum to bounce the bar off of and no shoulder capsule elasticity to help you drive the weight up. As exercises go, the overhead press is very pure.

Not so many years ago, the overhead press was one of the lifts contested in the sport of Olympic weightlifting alongside the snatch and clean and jerk. In an effort to hoist even larger weights, lifters leaned back to make the overhead press into a kind of standing incline press which made it hard to judge as well as being potentially dangerous. Subsequently, the standing overhead press, often referred to simply as the press, was dropped from Olympic lifting competitions in the early 1970's.

The overhead press is known by a number of names including shoulder press and military press but for simplicity, we'll use the term overhead press in this chapter, mainly to differentiate between this exercise and the bench press which was discussed in-depth earlier. The overhead press can be performed seated or standing, with dumbbells, barbell, kettlebells, sand bags or any other suitably heavy objects. We'll focus on the standing overhead barbell press in the main part of this chapter as it's the most effective and accessible form of the exercise but we'll take a look at these and other pressing variations later.

Overhead Press Anatomy

Pressing a weight overhead uses just about every muscle in your upper body with a particular emphasis on your deltoids or shoulder muscles and your triceps brachii which are the muscles on the back of your arm that extend your elbows. As the overhead press is performed in the standing position and without external support, your core muscles must work very hard to keep your spine correctly aligned and even your legs get in on the action as they support your upper body and the bar.

Commonly thought of as a shoulder exercise, the overhead press does place an emphasis on the anterior or front head of the tri-planar deltoids but the reality is the entire shoulder complex must work together to achieve the desired movement. Even the pectoralis major and latissimus dorsi muscles are strongly involved in the overhead press. If you only had time to perform one upper body exercise, you could do a lot worse than choosing the overhead press. Super-set with chin-ups and you have a very complete upper body workout in just two exercises. How's that for training efficiency?!

Pressing Equipment

The standing overhead press is best performed in a squat or power rack. This allows you to start the lift from a safe and comfortable position. You can clean the bar up to your shoulders but this a) uses valuable energy that is better spent pressing and b) requires that you can perform a good clean in the first place.

Clothing wise, anything will do so long as you are able to comfortably extend your arms above your head. Shoes are fairly important though and ideally you want a shoe with a solid and flat sole to minimize your risk of wobbling about. Running shoes are great for absorbing impact but the soles will distort when loaded heavily and so are not really recommended. If you don't have a suitable shoe, and your gym allows it, you might find that you are more stable if you remove your shoes lift in your socks. Mind your toes though!

As you'll be gripping the bar tightly, lifting chalk can be beneficial. If you don't have any or your gym forbids its use, dry your hands on a sweat towel before you start each set so you don't have to worry about your hands slipping.

Overhead Press Technique

Your initial set up is essential for good performance. Getting your starting position right increases your chances of lifting well from the outset. For the overhead press, the set up starts with making sure the bar is positioned at the right height in the rack...

Adjust the rack so that the bar is set at slightly below shoulder level. If your rack does not allow you to get the bar at exactly the right height, select a lower rather than higher setting. You can always dip your knees slightly to get yourself in a good lift off position whereas getting into a good lift off position on tip toes is never a good idea!

Once you have the bar at the right height, reach out and grip the bar with an overhand shoulder-width grip; ideally your forearms should be vertical when viewed from the front and your elbows directly below your hands.

Regarding your grip – while you should use a thumbs around grip for security, many lifters use a thumb-less grip when overhead pressing. Start by using a thumbs-around grip and then, once you have developed good pressing technique and have gained some confidence, progress to the thumb-less grip as necessary.

Walk toward the bar and position it at shoulder-height with your elbows below your hands as described above. Inhale, lift your chest, and use your legs to lift the bar clear of the hooks. Take a small step back and position your feet so they are between hip and shoulder-width apart.

Bend your knees slightly but then keep them absolutely still for the duration of your set. Your weight should be spread evenly from the balls of your feet to your heels. Make sure you can still wiggle your toes inside your shoes. If your weight shifts forwards onto your toes or backwards onto your heels, you are more likely to wobble and waste valuable energy correcting your posture. By making sure your weight is spread from the ball of your foot to your heel, you are more likely to keep the weight over your base of support.

Press your elbows slightly forwards and flair your lats Upper back muscles) as though you are trying to create a shelf for your arms to rest against. This action should help make your upper body more solid and provide a stable platform from which to press.

Exhale and inhale again so you start pressing with your lungs full of air. This will help stabilize your upper body. Brace your core muscles, lean back very slightly and then drive the bar straight up above your head. As the bar passes your face, lean forwards slightly so you are completely upright. This lean back and then forward manoeuvre is necessary so you don't hit your chin with the bar. Ideally, the bar should miss your chin and nose by an inch and not a mile!

Press the bar up to full arm extension but be careful not to hyperextend your elbows. There is a big difference between working through a full range of movement and snapping your elbows straight or beyond. The former is fine and encouraged while the latter should be avoided at all costs.

Lower the bar using the exact opposite path until it is back down to shoulder level. At this point, exhale, inhale, reset your core and repeat. It is common practice to exhale as you press the bar up but many disagree with this approach. Exhaling with your arms extended reduces intra-abdominal pressure just where you need it most – i.e. when the bar is the farthest away from your base of support, and will encourage your chest to drop. This is akin to slacking off the guide ropes on your tent just as the wind picks up! It's better to breathe between repetitions to maximize your core stability or, at the very least, inhale as you raise the bar and exhale as you lower it – the opposite of the breathing pattern prescribed by most trainers.

On completion of your set, walk forwards and re-rack the bar. Step away from the squat rack and congratulate yourself on a set well done.

Overhead Press Faults

Pressing a weight above your head sounds simple and, with practice, should feel perfectly natural but, like any exercise, there are some common faults to look out for.

- Avoid overextending or rounding your lower back. Doing so places an inordinate amount of pressure on your intervertebral discs. This problem may be caused by weak abdominals, overly tight hip flexors or hamstrings, too tight lats or pecs. If you have trouble maintaining perfect lower back posture while pressing, get a biomechanical assessment from a knowledgeable fitness professional who can pinpoint the problem. Also consider performing your presses using a supportive exercise bench.
- Keep your feet still. It's all too easy to move your feet between repetitions in an effort to try and gain some advantage that allows you to lift a little more weight or complete more repetitions. In actuality, all this achieves is wasting valuable energy. Imagine your feet are nailed to the floor so that they can provide the most solid platform possible. Keep your leg muscles tensed but still – your lower body must act like the bench in the bench press; solid and immovable.

- Do not use your legs to jerk the bar upwards. This is called a push press and while this is a legitimate exercise, as something to progress onto at a later date if you move into power training.
- Keep the bar level. It is not uncommon to have one arm stronger than the other. If you notice one arm is lagging behind, simply pull all of your mental energy into the weaker limb and you will probably find that you can keep the bar level more easily. Always limit your sets according to your weaker arm and stop as soon as your press becomes uneven. Eventually you will eliminate your left to right imbalances.
- Make sure your forearms are vertical to the floor. A wider or narrower hand position will cause your forearms to be angled outwards or inwards respectively. This makes your pushing action less efficient and may also place unnecessary stress on your wrists, elbows and shoulders. It's a question of mechanics.

Overhead Pressing Variations

The standing barbell overhead press is an excellent exercise but it's always nice to have a few alternatives to select from to keep your workouts fresh and interesting. Once you have mastered this exercise you may want to try some of these overhead pressing options. You'll notice that there is no mention of pressing using a Smith machine or pressing behind the neck. That is because both of these variations offer no real benefits and may actually cause you long term harm so stay clear of these two pressing options.

Seated Barbell Overhead Press

The standing overhead press is pretty much a whole body exercise but if you want to isolate your upper body from your lower body then seated presses are a good option. You can do this by simply sitting on the end of a flat exercise bench or using an upright exercise bench. The upright backrest provides support so all you have to do is concentrate on pushing the weight up above your head but at the cost of eliminating your core. On the downside, the path of the bar is slightly different as you have to move the bar around your head rather than your head around the bar is it travels up and down. Some lifters may find this feels less natural and places a potentially injurious stress on the shoulders. This can be avoided by using a very slightly inclined bench.

Dumbbell Presses

Using dumbbells requires more balance and coordination and also means that you can clean the weights up to shoulder level. If lifting as much weight as possible is your goal, stick with the barbell version but if you want to develop shoulder mass or general sports performance, dumbbells are a good choice. Perform dumbbells presses standing or seated, using one dumbbell at a time or two together.

Surfboard Presses

This fun pressing variation works your shoulders in a very unique way. Hold a dumbbell so that it is standing vertically in the palm of your hand at shoulder-level. Place your other hand on top. Press the dumbbell up and over your head so that it now rests on your opposite shoulder. The dumbbell should describe an arc as it travels over your head. Continue switching sides for the duration of your set. This exercise can be performed seated or standing.

Press from the Top

If you only have limited weight available but still want to work your shoulders hard, this exercise may be useful. Take a dumbbell in each hand and press them overhead to arms' length. Keep one arm extended and lower the opposite weight down to your shoulder. Press the weight back up and then lower the other weight. Continue to alternate sides while keeping one arm pressed to full extension the whole time. This keeps your shoulders under tension and will make even the lightest weight feel heavy after a few repetitions.

Bradford Press

Despite saying that pressing behind the neck is a bad idea, this limited range of movement exercise is okay if you have good shoulder and upper back mobility. If you have any doubt as to your suitability to this exercise, don't do it. Your shoulders are a relatively fragile joint and you'll miss them when they are gone so treat them with care! Performed with a barbell and in a seated or standing position, start with the bar in front of you at shoulder-height. Press the bar up and over so that it only just clears the top of your head. Lower the bar down to the back of your neck and then immediately press it up and over again. By eliminating the lockout, you keep the tension on your shoulder muscles and off your triceps. This is an effective mass building exercise but not really suitable in the pursuit of strength.

Bench presses might get the title of "most popular upper body exercise" but overhead pressing gets the title of "most beneficial". Work on your overhead press and your bench press numbers will soar and if you want shoulders like boulders, you have GOT to press!

Pull-up

The main problem with the pull up and chin up is that you have to be sufficiently strong to lift your entire bodyweight using the muscles of your upper body. While there are ways and means of reducing the amount of weight you have to lift, the fact remains that you need a reasonable level of strength to even perform these exercises. That raises the question, how to you get strong enough to do the exercise in the first place? As well as explaining how to perform these exercises, in this chapter we will provide you with a number of strategies that will help you achieve your first pull up/chin up and then subsequently improve you numbers.

Pull up and Chin up Anatomy

Pull ups are performed with an overhand slightly-wider than shoulder-width grip whereas chin ups use a narrower and underhand grip. Both exercises are comparable because although the shoulder movements are different, the muscles responsible for those movements are the same.

In pull ups, the arms are pulled downwards and into the midline of the body – a movement called shoulder adduction. In chin ups, the arms are pulled downward and backwards – a movement called shoulder extension.

Both adduction and extension are the job of your latissimus dorsi muscles, lats for short, which are located on the side of your back and, when well developed, resemble wings.

The main different between pull ups and chin ups is how the position of your hands affects the function of your elbows. In an overhand, also called a pronated grip, your biceps (the muscles on the front of your elbows and your primary elbow flexors) are in a mechanically disadvantageous position. Conversely, when you palms are facing towards you, also called a supinated grip, your biceps are in a stronger position and better able to generate force.

This means that pull ups are harder than chin ups so you may find simply performing the palms under version makes this exercise easier. Those of you already able to do five or more reps of pull ups can test this for yourself: Perform a set of pull ups to failure and then immediately switch to a supinated grip and amazingly you'll be able to complete a couple more reps as you move from a mechanically disadvantageous position to a more advantageous one.

Pull up and Chin up Equipment

You can perform these exercises on anything that safely allows you to hang at full stretch with your arms extended. There are specialist stations, often called power towers, designed for the sole purpose of doing pull ups and chin ups or you can hang from a power rack, Smith machine or even a sturdy roof beam or tree branch. So long as your feet are clear of the ground, anything will do the job.

As your grip is essential for good pull up/chin up performance, dry hands are a must so you might want to consider using lifting chalk or drying your hands on a towel before each set.

Some exercisers use webbing wrist straps or wrist hooks to enhance a weak grip however these straps merely address the symptom of weak forearms rather than providing a solution. If you do find your grip is a problem, by all means use wrist straps etc. but do your best to wean yourself off them so your grip gets stronger.

Pull up and Chin up Technique

Both these vertical pulling exercises are simple but that doesn't mean they are easy! Correct technique can help you avoid wasting energy and will make your movements more efficient and economical which should mean more repetitions performed...

Grasp a sturdy overhead bar with the appropriate grip – slightly wider than shoulder-width and palms facing away for pull ups or slightly narrower than shoulder-width and palms facing towards you for chin ups.

Hang from the bar with your arms extended. Bend your knees and cross your ankles – this helps to limit the amount of swinging you do under the bar which can break up your exercise rhythm.

Lift your chest and lean back slightly – the pull up and chin up are surprisingly tough on your core muscles so don't worry if you feel these muscles engaging as it's a good thing!

Pull smoothly but strongly with your arms. Continue pulling until your chin is ABOVE the bar and not just touching it. If you lean your head back and thrust your chin skywards you can probably touch the bar despite only performing three-quarters of a repetition so pull up and over and so cheating allowed.

Slowly extend your arms and lower yourself back to full arm extension but DO NOT relax your arms or shoulders between reps. Keep your muscles tense to protect your shoulder and elbow joints.

Chin up and Pull up Faults

Despite being a technically straight forward movement, it is still possible to make a hash of this effective but demanding exercise. Here are a few of the more common faults and how to fix them...

- **Failure to pull chin over the bar** – likely to be either a technical fault (poor exercise habits) or a biceps weakness. Try performing chin-ups instead of pull-ups, strengthening your biceps or using bands for assistance as described below
- **Failure to fully extend the arms at the bottom** – again, probably a technique fault so make a point of

pausing for a second with arms fully extended between repetitions to ensure this habit is eliminated. May also be a coping mechanism for making the reps easier by reducing range of movement. It's better to perform fewer reps using a full range of movement than more reps using a partial range of movement so no chopping your reps short as that is CHEATING!

- **Kicking with the legs** – sometimes called "kipping", using the legs can create a kind of "body wave" that helps you perform more repetitions by creating momentum. CrossFit, which often prescribes high repetitions of pull ups, use kipping quite a lot. If you are doing pull ups and chin ups for developmental purposes kipping is counterproductive as it merely takes stress off the target muscles of the lats and biceps. If, however, you are training for CrossFit then by all means add a kip but don't forget that strict pull ups and chin ups are your bread and butter in terms of muscular development.

- **Unable to do pull ups or chin ups** – don't worry as you are not alone! Here are some strategies below to help you do your first solo repetition and then increase your performance numbers...

Completing your first rep

Doing your first rep of pull ups or chin ups is a major fitness achievement and separates the boys from the men! Many exercisers go through life never achieving this goal and that's a shame as both the pull up and chin up are excellent upper body exercises. While on the subject of the genders, don't think for a minute that women can't do pull ups – they can!

As chin ups are the slightly easier of the two exercises, I suggest you start by concentrating on that variation and then progress to the pull up once you have begun to master the less demanding movement.

Assisted chin ups – if you are unable to lift your bodyweight, it makes sense that reducing your bodyweight will make the exercise easier to perform. This can be done in a couple of ways; you could use an assisted chin up machine where a weight is used to counterbalance your bodyweight. You could loop a strong resistance band over your chin up bar and then stand or kneel in the band so it provides some extra thrust or you could recruit the assistance of a strong spotter to help support some of your weight. Whichever method you choose, try to reduce the amount of assistance so that you get stronger. As you are training for strength, keep your reps below five and focus on quality over quantity.

Negative chin ups – while you might lack the strength to pull yourself up, you are probably strong enough to lower yourself down as your muscles are as much as 30% stronger as they lengthen. To do a negative chin up, climb up so your chin is over the bar and then slowly lower yourself down to full stretch. Immediately climb back up and repeat. When you are no longer able to control your descent, stop your set, rest a couple of minutes and then repeat.

Lock offs – it is quite common to hit a sticking point when performing chin ups at the point your elbows approach 90 degrees. This can be remedied by performing lock offs. Climb up and position your arms so they are bent to 90 degrees. Remove your feet and hold this position for as long as possible. Try to increase the length of your lock off over subsequent training sessions. With time, you should find you have no issue busting through this sticking point.

Strategies for Increasing your Reps

Once you can do more than a couple of reps, it's time to try and get your numbers up. These approaches can be applied to both pull ups and chin ups...

Little and often – a great way to increase your pull up or chin up numbers is to do lots of sets of low reps throughout your workout. For example, if you can do three reps, perform lots of sets of one rep. Do a set of pull ups or chin ups in between each set of your other exercises so by the end of your workout you will have performed as many as 20 sub-maximal sets. With this method, it is essential you always keep a rep or two in reserve and do not go to failure. To learn to do a lot of pull ups you need to do a lot of pull ups and that means avoiding failure and focusing on quality reps.

Ladders – a ladder is a broken set made up of mini sets called rungs. Perform one repetition, rest a moment, then perform two reps, rest again, three reps, rest, and so on. When you can't reach the next "rung" of your workout, take an extended rest and then start over at one. This is a great way of increasing exercise volume as if you manage a ladder of one/two/three repetitions, you will have actually completed six repetitions when, quite likely, you'd only manage four reps using a more traditional rep/set scheme.

Weighted – One of the best methods for increasing my pull up numbers is increasing pull up strength. Strap a weight around your waist or put on a weighted vest and perform four to six weeks of low rep strength training – no more than five reps per set. When you next perform a set of regular bodyweight pull ups, you will have a greater amount of strength and this will make the exercise easier so you'll be able to more reps. Take care though, the added weight can place a lot of stress on your elbows and shoulders so make sure you use perfect technique.

Pull up and chin up Variations

Try these pull up and chin up variations to add some spice to your workouts!

Towel grip pull ups

Loop two hand towels over your pull up bar and grab the ends tightly. Perform your pull ups as normal. This variation is an awesome gripping exercise and ideal for climbers and grapplers.

Climber pull ups

Position your hands as for regular pull ups put instead of pulling your chin up to the centre of the bar, pull yourself up and over so your chin touches your left hand. Return to the start position and then pull up to the right. For a harder version, pull up to the left and then keep your chin above the bar and traverse across to your right hand before lowering. Reverse your direction of travel for the next rep.

Mixed grip pull ups

Using a shoulder-width grip, place one hand in a pronated position and the other in a supinated position. Make sure you swap hands set by set.

Sternum pull ups

Using a V grip bar or single towel, hang beneath the bar so your body is turned through 90 degrees. Pull up and simultaneously lean back so your sternum touches the bar and not your chin. This places a large emphasis on your middle trapezius and rhomboid muscles in the centre of your back. Be aware that the excessive spinal extension can place a lot of stress on your back so use this variation with caution.

Doing chin-ups and pull-ups really separates the men from the boys and is worthy of a nod of acknowledgement from most other gym-users. Not only are chin-ups and pull-ups great back builders, they are also a terrific biceps

builder too. Broader back and bigger arms; what's not to love about chin-ups and pull-ups!

Conclusion

So, know you have a great workout to follow and some detailed instructions as to how you should perform the most effective muscle building exercises around so you are all set, right? Not so fast buddy!

Training is very important but training alone won't get you strong and muscular. You also have to consider your diet and your lifestyle too…

Diet

Just as you cannot build a house without bricks, you can't build muscle without food. Food provides your body with both energy and the material it needs for making your muscles bigger and stronger. As good as this programme is, it won't work unless you give your body all the food it needs. Here are a few diet tips to ensure you are not inadvertently sabotaging your progress…

- Eat frequently – frequent meals ensure your body gets a steady supply of nutrients which is essential for muscle growth
- Hydrate – your body needs at least two litres of water per day so make sure you drink little and often
- Protein – you need around1.2 and 1.8 grams of protein per kilo of bodyweight so make sure mny of your meals include protein. Consider using a protein supplement if you are unable to eat enough legumes, seeds, nuts, whole grains etc. (whole food plant based diet; I am not a big fan of animal based protein)
- If you aren't gaining weight, eat more – if you are training hard and still not getting the results you want, increase your food intake. Add an extra meal or couple of snacks per day until you start to see improvements

- Eat healthily – a bodybuilding diet should be, by definition, a healthy diet rich in vitamins and minerals and low in sugar are artificial additives. The healthier you are, the better your body will be able to build muscle

Lifestyle

As well as training and diet, your lifestyle also plays a big part in your bodybuilding success...

- Get 8+ hours of sleep – your muscles recover and grow not when you exercise but when you sleep so make sure you are getting enough
- Minimize stress – stress produces a muscle-destroying hormone called cortisol so keep your stress levels low for best muscle-building results
- Go easy on the cardio – cardio might be good for your health but too much can rob your body of essential energy and limit your results. If you are serious about gaining muscle you would do well to limit your cardio to no more than one hour per week
- Train with intensity – leave your phone in your locker and don't stop at the water cooler to chat to your buddies. Go the gym to work – not relax. Muscles are resistant to change so you'll need to work hard if you want to see the best possible results
- Consider the impact smoking and drinking alcohol will have on your results – both smoking and excess alcohol consumption will hinder your training results because both will have a negative effect on your health. Be like the golden age bodybuilders – be healthy AND be strong.

Building muscle and developing strength are seldom easy but that's why building muscle is such a rewarding activity – nothing worth achieving ever comes without effort. If you commit to the process, are determined and persistent, you will achieve great things and every kilo of muscle you build will be your reward. So, dig in and work hard – you CAN do it!